The Easy L Instant Pot Cookbook for Beginners

Healthy & Tasty Lectin Free Recipes for Instant Pot Pressure Cooker

Emmanuel Lawrence

Copyright © 2018 by Emmanuel Lawrence

All rights reserved worldwide.

ISBN: 978-1722908270

You may not reproduce or transmitte any part of the book, in any form or by any means, electronic or mechanical, including photocopying, recording or by any information storage and retrieval system, without written permission from the publisher or author, except for the inclusion of brief quotations in a review.

Warning-Disclaimer

The purpose of this book is to educate and entertain. The author or publisher does not guarantee that anyone following the techniques, suggestions, tips, ideas, or strategies will become successful. The author and publisher shall have neither liability or responsibility to anyone with respect to any loss or damage caused, or alleged to be caused, directly or indirectly by the information contained in this book.

Contents

Introduction 4

Soups 12
Spinach Soup 12
Chicken Broth with Broccoli 12
Turkey Mixed Soup Recipe 13
Mushroom Soup Recipe 14
Chicken and Kale Soup 14
Vegetable Soup 15

Pork and Beef 16
Creamy Pork in a Mushroom and Root Beer Sauce 16
Pork Butt with Mushrooms and Celery 16
Pork Chops with Brussel Sprouts 17
Braised Red Cabbage and Bacon 18
Apple Cider Pork Shoulder 18
Lectin Free Ground Pork with Cabbage 19
Ground Pork and Sauerkraut 20
Sage Pork Butt and Yams 20
Pork Meatloaf with Ketchup 21
Tangy Pork in a Tomato and Sour Cream Sauce 22
Pork Meatballs in an Lemon Juice Sauce 23
Pork Steaks with Apple and Apricot 23
Pork Sausage with Sweet Onions 24
Rosemary Dijon Apple Pork 25

Smothered Cinnamon BBQ Ribs	25
Pork Ribs and Pearl Onions Under Pressure	26
Barbecue Pork Butt	27
Pork with Rutabaga and Granny Smith Apples	28
Spicy Ground Pork	28
Pork Chops in Merlot	29
Pork Chops and Mushrooms in a Tomato Sauce	30
Braised Chili Pork Chops	31
Beef Cabbage Rolls in a Tomato Sauce	32
Beef Ribs with Button Mushrooms	32
Beef Medley with Blue Cheese Roquefort and Cabbage	33
Basil and Thyme Pot Roast	34
Worcestershire Beef Brisket	35
Beef in a Creamy Sour Sauce	35
Ground Beef, Leek, and Sauerkraut	36
Corned Beef in a Celery Sauce	37
Beef Sausage and Red Cabbage Casserole	38
Drunken Beef and Mushrooms	38
Dark Beer and Dijon Braised Steak	39
Tender Onion Beef Roast	40
Spicy Shredded Beef	41
Teriyaki and Peach Pulled Beef	42
Sweet Balsamic Beef	42
Marinated Flank Steak	43
Bourbon and Apricot Meatloaf	44
Herbed Beef Cubes	45
Simple Cheesy Meatballs	45

Coconut Beef with Plantains 46

Mexican Brisket 47

Poultry 48

Chicken in Beer Sauce 48

Balsamic Chicken Thighs with Mango 48

Lectin Free Coconut Milk Chicken 49

Sweet and Gingery Whole Chicken 50

Habanero Turkey Breasts 51

Cranberry Turkey Wings 51

Curry and Coconut Milk Chicken 52

Mustard and Lime Goose 53

Turkey Meatloaf 53

Balsamic Chicken 54

Simple Garlicky Goose 55

Thyme and Lemon Drumsticks 55

Smoked Paprika Chicken Legs 56

Bacon and Cheese Shredded Chicken 57

Mexican Turkey Breasts 58

Garlic and Thyme Chicken 58

Basil and Oregano Duck Breasts 59

Vegetable and Side Dishes 60

Prosciutto Collards 60

Buttery Golden Beets 60

Cauliflower and Egg Salad 61

Broccoli Cheese 61

Rutabaga and Scallion Side 62

Lime and Mayo Steamed Broccoli 63

Zesty Onions 63

Lemony Brussel Sprouts 64

Balsamic Caper Beets 64

Tamari Bok Choy 65

Creamy Goat Cheese Cauliflower 66

Frascati and Sage Broccoli 66

Sweet Caramelized Onions 67

Turmeric Kale with Shallots 67

Snacks & Appetizers 69

Buttery Beets 69

Cheese and Polenta Balls 69

Sheep Cheese Veggie Appetizer 70

Mini Beefy Cabbage Rolls 71

Southern Chicken Dip 71

Minty Grape Leaves 72

Hardboiled Eggs 73

Salmon Bites 74

Chili Sriracha Eggs 74

Tempeh Sandwiches 75

Chef's Selection 76

Chicken Liver Pate 76

Eggs de Provence 76

Whole Hog Omelet 77

Veal and Mushrooms 78

Cheese and Prosciutto Eggs 78

Easy Duck with and Ginger 79
Buttery and Lemony Dill Clams 80
Pork Liver and Spring Onion Pate 80
Vegan Holiday Roast 81
Hassle-Free Holiday Roast 81
Quail and Pancetta 82
White Wine Mussels 83
Party Duck Bites 84
Festive Rosemary Chicken 84
Party Crab Legs 85
Fancy Shrimp Scampi 86

Introduction

It's no secret that the Instant Pot is a total game-changer when it comes to healthy eating. Where healthy eating once took a lot of time and energy, this fun gadget lets you cook a better-for-you meal in minutes. People who follow all sorts of healthy diets have found an easier way to cook using their Instant Pot. The creators of the Instant Pot have made this device extremely user-friendly, so virtually anyone can get started.

If you're short on time, you are going to appreciate the Instant Pot. Where you once had to waste your precious time chopping veggies to just the right size and defrosting meat for an hour before you could even start to cook it, you're now completely free to spend minimal time in the kitchen. In fact, the Instant Pot does most of the work for you. My favorite thing about Instant Pot cooking is the ability to create gourmet-tasting meals in the time it takes to go to the drive-thru and back. There's no excuse to not create the health of your dreams!

This is My First Instant Pot!

If you're new to the Instant Pot circle, let me welcome you in with this brief overview: The Instant Pot is a high-tech pressure cooker that replaces quite a few of your kitchen appliances. You can throw out your slow cooker, old pressure cooker, vegetable steamer and even your yogurt maker. The Instant Pot works by using liquid to create steam, which in turn creates high-pressure that cooks food extremely fast. For instance, you can have a cup of rice cooked in five minutes or less.

The Instant Pot is great for people with busy lifestyles because it not only cuts your cooking time down, but you have no need to check on what your cooking every few minutes. It also cuts your prep time down because you can cook things straight from the freezer. No need to waste time defrosting meat! Bonus: You don't have to wash a whole sink of dishes every time you eat! Your kitchen will look a lot cleaner and your wallet will thank you for not purchasing the latest and greatest cooking device to complement your healthy eating plan.

Best of all? Your food won't lose valuable vitamins and minerals like it would with other cooking methods. This is because you're not drowning your food in water, but rather giving it just enough liquid to create the perfect amount of steam. Your meat stays tender and your vegetables remain crisp using this cooking method. You'll wow your friends and create healthy meals that you'll be excited to eat. I love how much flavor my lectin-free Instant Pot meals have! The Instant Pot is simply amazing and one of my most used kitchen tools. Trust me when I say it will be your new best friend.

Why Follow a Lectin-Free Diet?

Simply put, lectin-free diets avoid lectins as much as possible. Lectins are a type of protein that's found in a lot of plant-based foods, particularly whole grains, beans and, legumes. Plants use these lectins to avoid being eaten by insects. Many people choose to avoid lectins because they can cause anything from stomach issues to increased risk of chronic illness. Many people have claimed that following a lectin-free diet has helped them decrease inflammation, lose weight and even boost their mood. If you're someone who struggles with "leaky gut" issues or if you're struggling to lose weight, this is a less invasive option you'll want to consider.

Some dieters avoid all foods that contain lectin, but following a lectin-free diet doesn't necessarily mean avoiding these foods altogether. It does mean that you're actively working to decrease the lectins in the food you consume. Slow cooking, boiling, and roasting lectin-filled foods aren't recommended by health professionals because the temperature isn't high enough to successfully eliminate lectins, but pressure cooking (what your Instant Pot does!) has been proven to effectively decrease lectins. Many dieters are even recommending soaking your beans and legumes before pressure cooking them.

Lectin-Free diets focus on the following foods:

- Pasture-raised meats
- Sweet potatoes
- Green, leafy vegetables like kale and spinach
- Cruciferous Vegetables (Broccoli, Brussels sprouts)
- Garlic
- Celery
- Avocado
- Mushrooms
- Olives
- Extra virgin olive oil

- Nuts and seeds
- Millet
- Wild-caught fish

If you're trying to eliminate lectins in your food, you'll likely want to rarely consume foods like:

- Beans, lentils, peanuts (Unless properly cooked, ex: Pressure cooking)
- Squash
- Nightshade vegetables (tomatoes, potatoes, peppers)
- Fruit (Except in moderation!)
- Grains
- Dairy

You'll definitely want to avoid eating:

- Corn
- Meat from corn-fed animals
- A1 milk

Ditch and Switch: Stock your pantry with these items!

When converting to a lectin-free diet, you'll want to make sure you have the following things on hand. The most budget-conscious way to replace items is to gradually replace them with a better option when you run out. You have to purchase a new item anyway, might as well make it one that fits with your healthy lifestyle! Here are my pantry must-haves:

- Iodized or fine sea salt
- Extra virgin olive oil
- Avocado oil
- Balsamic vinegar

- Arrowroot starch
- Flours like Cassava, Almond, and Coconut
- Ground flax seed
- Dark Chocolate (75 % and above!)
- Pure vanilla extract
- Coconut Milk
- Sweeteners like monk fruit, honey and,erythritol
- Indian Basmati rice
- Shirataki noodles
- Flax-seed crackers
- Seeds (Hemp or flax)
- White almond butter
- Vegetable and mushroom broths
- Sweet potato puree
- Canned wild salmon
- Toasted sesame oil
- Tahini
- Nuts like macadamia or pistachios

Why Did I Write This Cookbook?

As a follower of a lectin-free diet, it was hard to find recipes that used my most convenient kitchen device; the Instant Pot. I found many recipes online for baking and even a few that contained cooking methods that aren't recommended for reducing lectins. Furthermore, many of the recipes I came across didn't look like things your average diner would eat in an emergency, much less every day. I knew there was a way to create lectin-free food that brings joy to your life! I wanted to create a cookbook that would give healthy eaters delicious food that wouldn't take long to cook. I wanted to give you family-friendly meals that you can pull together without sacrificing your family-time. I believe that everyone deserves the right to have healthy meals that fit in with their healthy eating convictions. Creating recipes that used an Instant Pot was a no-brainer. With pressure cooking being the most recommended way for lectin-free people to prepare food, these recipes would combine ease with optimal health benefits.

I wrote this cookbook to make your life easier and more enjoyable. To give you the stress-free healthy eating plan you crave. I know firsthand that when you eat food that makes you feel good, your energy goes up, your mood improves and the rest of your life slowly falls into place. I hope that this can be the first of many baby steps you take on your journey to better health and I'm proud to be apart of it!

What Can I Expect From This Cookbook?

In this cookbook, you'll find many delicious recipes that will help you eliminate lectins from your diet in an easy way. Whether you're a Mom on the go or an office executive, life gets busy. You shouldn't have to sacrifice your health convictions for your schedule. I can't tell you how many times my Instant Pot has saved me from making a not-so-wise choice at the drive-thru!

These recipes don't require a lot of prep, but they may involve some ingredients you need to invest in. These ingredients will become well-loved staples in your lectin-free kitchen, so think of this as an investment in your health. The recipes are written in a concise, easy to understand way. I tried to make my directions as clear as possible because no one likes over complicated instructions!

My Best Instant Pot Tips and Tricks for YOUR Success!

Using an Instant Pot isn't nearly as hard as it seems. Here are my best hacks to help you get the best results with each recipe in this cookbook.

- Read your instruction manual. Each Instant Pot is different and has different features and needs.
- Quick pressure release means that you're using the knob on the top of your Instant Pot to quickly release the steam pressure.
- Natural pressure release is simply letting the pressure decrease by itself. This takes more time than quick pressure release.
- It's important to follow the directions of each recipe for either "quick release or natural release". This ensures that the recipe cools down at the correct speed.
- If you're using your Instant Pot for every meal, you may want to purchase an extra stainless steel sleeve. This helps you to always have a spare on hand when the other is dirty.
- If you're cooking a whole, frozen cut of meat try using the trivet that comes with most Instant Pots. This will help your meat to cook evenly.
- Remember, the Instant Pot is extremely safe and nothing to be scared of. It can seem intimidating at first to start cooking in this way, but take it slow follow directions and you'll get the hang of it!
- Be sure to use a pot-holder or oven mitt when handling a hot Instant Pot. Many Instant Pots come with silicone mitts that will protect your hands.
- The Instant Pot works best for foods that you would normally cook in your slow-cooker. You won't get a crispy pizza crust with this method, but you can sure cook a mean pot-roast!
- Keep children away from the Instant Pot while it's in use.
- Make sure you're using enough liquid when steaming your veggies! Your Instant Pot needs a certain amount of liquid to rev up!

- Don't overfill your Instant Pot. A good rule of thumb is to only fill it to the fill line. You'll find this line on the inside of your stainless steel sleeve.
- You can delay your cooking to start your Instant Pot at the time that's best for you or to keep your meal warm. This is one of the best features, in my opinion!
- Cleaning your Instant Pot correctly will ensure that it lasts a long time! I recommend cleaning most parts in the dishwasher, as that's fast and effective. Don't have a dishwasher? You can break down mineral deposits using vinegar or lemon juice.
- To get stubborn odors (hello garlic!) out of your instant pot, you can steam water and lemon wedges.
- When choosing your Instant Pot, take into consideration the size of your family! There's nothing worse than not being able to fit your ingredients in your pot!

On an Ending Note

I hope you enjoy this cookbook! I know that it will soon become one of your favorite resources for following a lectin-free diet. If you're just starting to follow this way of eating, I want to encourage you that it is possible to find joy in what you're cooking. The Instant Pot makes meat tender, veggies crisp and flavorful and it brings an ease to your life that can be hard to find when eating healthy. You'll find there really isn't anything your Instant Pot can't cook for you!

My greatest hope is that this cookbook will inspire you to not only use the recipes found within its pages but that you'd find a spark of creativity and create some of your own lectin-free concoctions.

Happy Cooking!

Soups

Spinach Soup

(Prep + Cook Time: 35 minutes / Servings: 4)

Ingredients:

- 4 cups Vegetable broth
- 1 cup Baby Spinach
- 2 Garlic cloves, minced
- ½ cup Coconut Milk
- 2 tablespoons Olive oil
- 1 cup Organic Heavy cream
- 1 bunch Coriander, puree
- ½ teaspoon Chili flakes
- ¼ teaspoon Salt

Directions:

1. Heat oil and add garlic cloves, cook for 1 minute on SAUTÉ mode.
2. Add vegetable broth, spinach, coriander puree, cream, chili flake, and salt, mix well.
3. Close the lid and cook on SOUP mode for 30 minutes.
4. Once cooking is complete, allow pressure to release naturally for 10 minutes, then set steam vent to Venting to quick-release remaining pressure.
5. Pour in coconut milk and cook for 5 minutes on low heat.
6. Spoon into serving bowls and enjoy.

Chicken Broth with Broccoli

(Prep + Cook Time: 25 minutes / Servings: 4)

Ingredients:

- 1 package Broccoli, frozen
- 4 cups Chicken broth

- ½ cup Ghee Butter
- 1 Onion, chopped
- 1 tbsp. Garlic powder
- ½ cup Xanthan Gum
- 1 cup Water

Directions:

1. Add butter and onion into the Cooking pot. Press SAUTÉ and stir-fry for a minute.
2. Add in the xanthan gum, water, garlic powder, broccoli and chicken broth.
3. Press SOUP at high pressure and cook for 45 minutes.
4. When ready, do a quick pressure release and strain the stock.
5. Transfer the stock into containers and freeze up to 2 months.

Turkey Mixed Soup Recipe

(Prep + Cook Time: 30 minutes / Servings: 4)

Ingredients:

- 3 cups Turkey breast, cubed
- 4 cups Chicken broth
- 4 stalks Celery, chopped
- 2 Garlic cloves
- 1 Onion, chopped
- 2 cups Green onions, chopped
- Salt and pepper, to taste

Directions:

1. Add all ingredients to the Pot and stir well.
2. Seal the lid on the Instant Pot. Cook on SOUP at high pressure for 30 minutes.
3. Once complete, and the pressure released quickly, set aside to cool for 20 minutes before serving. Ladle into bowls garnish with green onions.

Mushroom Soup Recipe

(Prep + Cook Time: 40 minutes / Servings: 4)

Ingredients:

- 4 cups Chicken stock
- 4 cups Mushrooms, chopped
- 2 cups Sheep Sheese, shredded
- 2 tbsp. Ghee Butter
- 2 Onions, chopped
- 2 tbsp. Coconut Flour
- 2 Garlic cloves
- 1 cup Thyme, chopped

Directions:

1. Heat butter and add in the onions into the pot and stir-fry on SAUTÉ mode for 1 minute. Add in mushrooms, garlic, thyme, and chicken stock. Stir to combine.
2. Close the lid and select SOUP at high pressure for 25 minutes. Once ready, do a quick pressure relaese and open the lid.
3. Add the flour and let it simmer for 15 minutes on SLOW cook mode.
4. Sprinkle with shredded cheese and serve!

Chicken and Kale Soup

(Prep + Cook Time: 30 minutes / Servings: 4)

Ingredients:

- 1 lb. Chicken thighs, cubed
- 3 cups Chicken broth
- 2 cups Kale, chopped
- 2 tbsp. Olive oil
- Salt and pepper

Directions:

1. Heat oil in the Instant Pot on SAUTÉ mode. Add in chicken broth, kale, chicken cubes, salt and pepper.
2. Press SOUP and cook at high pressure for 25 minutes. Once ready, immediately turn steam vent to Venting to Quick Release pressure.
3. Ladle soup into individual bowls and serve.

Vegetable Soup

(Prep + Cook Time: 30 minutes / Servings: 4)

Ingredients:

- 1 cup Broccoli florets
- 1 cup Cabbage, shredded
- 3 cups Vegetable broth
- 1 Onion, sliced
- 2 Garlic cloves, minced
- 1 tablespoon Lemon juice
- ½ teaspoon Black pepper
- ¼ teaspoon Salt
- 1 tablespoon Cooking oil

Directions:

1. Set the Instant Pot on SAUTÉ mode.
2. Heat oil, add onion and garlic cloves, and stir-fry for 1 minute. Add in all the vegetables, stir-fry and cook for 8-10 minutes.
3. Add in the vegetable broth, salt, and pepper and mix well.
4. Close the lid and press SOUP. Adjust the cooking time to 25 minutes.
5. Once ready, do a quick release, drizzle lemon juice and ladle into serving bowls.

Pork and Beef

Creamy Pork in a Mushroom and Root Beer Sauce

(Prep + Cook Time: 50 minutes / Servings: 8)

Ingredients:

- 3 pounds Pork Roast
- 8 ounces Mushroom, sliced
- 12 ounces Root Beer
- 10 ounces Cream of Mushroom Soup
- 1 package of Dry Onion Soup
- ½ bunch parsley leaves, chopped to garnish

Directions:

1. Whisk together the mushroom soup, dry onion soup mix, and root beer in the Instant Pot. Add the mushrooms and pork.
2. Close the lid and set to MEAT/STEW mode. Cook for 40 minutes at high pressure.
3. Let sit for 5 minutes before doing a quick pressure release. Sprinkle with fresh parsley and serve.

Pork Butt with Mushrooms and Celery

(Prep + Cook Time: 35 minutes / Servings: 4)

Ingredients:

- 1 pound Pork Butt, sliced
- 2 cups sliced Mushrooms
- 1 ½ cup chopped Celery Stalk
- ⅓ cup White Wine
- 1 tsp minced Garlic
- ½ cup Chicken Broth
- Salt and Pepper to taste
- ½ bunch cilantro leaves, chopped to garnish

Directions:

1. Coat your Instant Pot with some cooking spray and heat to SAUTÉ.
2. Add the pork slices and cook for 4-5 minutes until browned.
3. Add mushrooms and celery and stir in the remaining ingredients.
4. Press MEAT/STEW and close the lid. Cook for 20 minutes at high pressure.
5. Release the pressure naturally for 10 minutes. Garnish with cilantro before serving.

Pork Chops with Brussel Sprouts

(Prep + Cook Time: 30 minutes / Servings: 4)

Ingredients:

- 4 Pork Chops
- ½ pound Brussel Sprouts
- ⅓ cup Sparkling Wine
- 1 ½ cups Beef Stock
- 2 Shallots, chopped
- 1 tbsp Olive Oil
- 1 cup chopped Celery Stalk
- 1 tbsp Coriander
- ¼ tsp Salt
- ¼ tsp Pepper
- 2 green onions, finely sliced to garnish

Directions:

1. Heat the olive oil in your Instant Pot on SAUTÉ. Add the pork chops and cook until browned on all sides. Stir in the remaining ingredients.
2. Select MEAT/STEW, close the lid and cook for 15 minutes at high pressure.
3. When the cooking cycle ends, allow pressure to natural release for 10 minutes. Transfer brussels sprouts to a plate with pork chops.
4. Garnish with green onions and serve immediately.

Braised Red Cabbage and Bacon

(Prep + Cook Time: 20 minutes / Servings: 8)

Ingredients:

- 1 pound Red Cabbage, chopped
- 8 Bacon Slices, chopped
- 1 ½ cups Beef Broth
- 2 tbsp Ghee Butter
- ½ tsp Salt and pepper
- ½ a bunch of fresh flat-leaf parsley to garnish

Directions:

1. Add the bacon slices in your Instant Pot, set it to SAUTÉ, and cook for 5 minutes, or until crispy.
2. Stir in the cabbage, salt, pepper, and butter. Seal the lid and cook on MANUAL for 10 minutes.
3. Use quick the release valve to release pressure. Scoop into a serving dish and sprinkle over the parsley, then serve.

Apple Cider Pork Shoulder

(Prep + Cook Time: 50 minutes / Servings: 4)

Ingredients:

- 1 pound Pork Shoulder
- ⅓ cup Apple Cider
- ¾ cup Water
- 3 tsp Olive Oil
- 1 tsp Cayenne Pepper
- 1 tbsp Sesame Oil
- Salt and Pepper, to taste

Directions:

1. Heat the oil in your Instant Pot on SAUTÉ. Season the pork with cayenne pepper, salt, and pepper.

2. Add to the Instant Pot and sear on all sides for a few minutes. Stir in the remaining ingredients.
3. Close the lid, select MANUAL and cook for 40 minutes.
4. Release the pressure naturally for 10 minutes. Transfer the pork to a platter and drizzle some of sauce over.

Lectin Free Ground Pork with Cabbage

(Prep + Cook Time: 25 minutes / Servings: 6)

Ingredients:

- 1 ⅓ pounds Ground Pork
- 1 cup shredded Cabbage
- ½ cup chopped Celery
- 2 Red Onions, chopped
- 1 Carrot, shredded
- 1 Bell Pepper, chopped
- ⅓ tsp Cumin
- 1 tsp Red Pepper Flakes
- Salt and Pepper, to taste

Directions:

1. Coat the Instant Pot with cooking spray and cook the ground pork until browned on SAUTÉ. Stir in the remaining ingredients.
2. Select MEAT/STEW, close the lid and cook for 15 minutes at high pressure.
3. Allow the pressure to release naturally for 10 minutes.
4. Transfer to a serving plate and serve alone or over cauliflower rice.

Ground Pork and Sauerkraut

(Prep + Cook Time: 25 minutes / Servings: 6)

Ingredients:

- 1 ¼ pounds Ground Pork
- 4 cups shredded Sauerkraut
- 1 cup Tomato Puree from deseeded / peeled tomatoes
- ½ cup Chicken Stock
- 1 Red Onion, chopped
- 2 Garlic Cloves, minced
- 2 Bay Leaves
- Salt and Pepper, to taste

Directions:

1. Set to SAUTÉ and brown the ground pork about 4-5 minutes.
2. Add the onions, garlic and cook until they are soft, about 2-3 minutes.
3. Stir in the remaining ingredients and season with salt and pepper. Choose MEAT/STEW, close the lid and cook for 15 minutes at high pressure.
4. When the cooking cycle ends, allow pressure to natural release for 10 minutes. Open the lid, remove the bay leaves and serve warm.

Sage Pork Butt and Yams

(Prep + Cook Time: 20 minutes / Servings: 4)

Ingredients:

- 1 pound Pork Butt, cut into 4 equal pieces
- 1 pound Yams, diced
- 2 tsp Ghee Butter
- ¼ tsp Thyme
- 1 ½ tsp Sage
- 1 ½ cups Beef Broth
- Salt and Pepper, to taste
- cilantro leaves, to garnish

Directions:

1. Season the pork with thyme, sage, salt, and pepper.
2. Melt the butter in your Instant Pot on SAUTÉ.
3. Add the pork and sear on all sides until brown, about 3-4 minutes per side. Add the yams and pour the broth over.
4. Select MEAT/STEW, close the lid and cook for 15 minutes at high pressure.
5. Allow the pressure to release naturally, for at least 10 minutes.
6. Remove the lid and taste; adjust seasoning if necessary. Garnish with cilantro before serving.

Rosemary Dijon Apple Pork

(Prep + Cook Time: 60 minutes / Servings: 6)

Ingredients:

- 3 ½ pounds Pork Roast
- 2 Apples, peeled and slices
- 3 tbsp Dijon Mustard
- 1 tbsp dried Rosemary
- ½ cup White Wine
- 1 tbsp minced Garlic
- 1 tbsp Oil
- Salt and Pepper, to taste
- 1 tbsp chopped fresh parsley

Directions:

1. Brush the mustard over the pork.
2. Heat the oil in your Instant Pot on SAUTÉ and sear the pork on all sides, about 3-4 minutes per side. Add apples and stir in the remaining ingredients.
3. Select MEAT/STEW, close the lid and cook for 40 minutes at high pressure. Release the pressure naturally for 10 minutes.
4. Serve pork warm, sprinkled with parsley.

Pork Meatballs in an Lemon Juice Sauce

(Prep + Cook Time: 30 minutes / Servings: 8)

Ingredients:

- 2 ½ pounds ground Pork
- ¼ cup Tamari Sauce
- 3 Garlic Cloves, minced
- ½ tbsp dried Thyme
- ½ cup diced Onions
- 2 tsp Honey
- ¼ cup Lemon Juice
- 1 ½ cups Water
- 1 cup Pork Rinds
- Salt and Pepper, to taste
- Zest of one lemon, to garnish

Directions:

1. Whisk together the honey, tamari, apple juice, water, and thyme in the Instant Pot. Season with salt and pepper.
2. Choose the MEAT/STEW mode and cook for 10 minutes at high pressure.
3. Meanwhile, combine all the remaining ingredients in a bowl.
4. Shape meatballs out of the mixture.
5. Release the pressure naturally for 10 minutes and drop the meatballs into the sauce.
6. Close the lid and cook on POULTRY for 15 minutes.
7. When the cooking cycle ends, allow pressure to natural release for 10 minutes.
8. Serve meatballs with the sauce poured over and garnished with lemon zest curls.

Pork Meatloaf with Ketchup

(Prep + Cook Time: 70 minutes / Servings: 4)

Ingredients:

- 1 pound ground Sausage
- 1 pound ground Pork
- ¾ cup Coconut Milk
- ½ tsp Cayenne Powder
- ½ tsp Marjoram
- 2 Eggs, beaten
- 2 Garlic Cloves, minced
- 1 Onion, diced

Topping:

- 1 cup Ketchup homemade from deseeded / peeled tomatoes

Directions:

1. Place all of the meatloaf ingredients in a bowl and mix with your hands to combine.
2. Grease the Instant Pot with cooking spray. Press the meatloaf mixture into the cooker.
3. Top with the ketchup. Close the lid and cook on MEAT/STEW for 60 minutes at high pressure.
4. When the cooking cycle ends, allow pressure to natural release for 10 minutes
5. Cool for 10 mins, then drain off any excess liquid and turn out onto a board. Cut into thick slices and serve warm with salad.

Tangy Pork in a Tomato and Sour Cream Sauce

(Prep + Cook Time: 45 minutes / Servings: 6)

Ingredients:

- 1 ½ pounds Pork Shoulder cut into pieces
- 2 Onions, chopped
- 1 ½ cups Sour Cream
- 1 cup Tomato Puree from deseeded / peeled tomatoes.
- ½ tbsp Coriander
- ¼ tsp Cumin
- ¼ tsp Cayenne Pepper
- 1 tsp minced Garlic
- Salt and Pepper, to taste

Directions:

1. Coat the Instant Pot with some cooking spray and brown the pork on SAUTÉ. Add onions and garlic and cook for 2-3 minutes.
2. Stir in the remaining ingredients and close the lid.
3. Select MEAT/STEW and cook for 30 minutes at high pressure.
4. When the cooking cycle ends, allow pressure to natural release for 10 minutes. Serve warm.

Pork Sausage with Sweet Onions

(Prep + Cook Time: 25 minutes / Servings: 8)

Ingredients:

- 8 Pork Sausages
- 2 large Sweet Onions, sliced
- ½ cup Beef Broth
- ¼ cup White Wine
- 1 tsp minced Garlic

Directions:

1. Set to SAUTÉ and brown the sausages. Transfer to a plate and discard the liquid. Heat the oil and stir-fry the onions for 2 minutes.
2. Stir in the garlic and sausages. Pour over the broth and wine. Close the lid and cook on MANUAL for 10 minutes.
3. When the cooking cycle ends, allow pressure to release naturally for 10 minutes. Serve immediately.

Smothered Cinnamon BBQ Ribs

(Prep + Cook Time: 85 minutes / Servings: 4)

Ingredients:

- 3 pounds Pork Ribs
- ½ cup Apple Jelly
- 1 cup Barbecue Sauce
- 1 Onion, diced
- 2 tbsp ground Cloves
- ½ cup Water
- 1 tbsp Stevia Brown Sugar
- 1 tsp Worcestershire Sauce
- 1 tsp ground Cinnamon

Directions:

1. Whisk together all the ingredients in your Instant Pot.
2. Place the ribs inside and close the lid.
3. Set the cooker to MEAT/STEW and cook for 60 minutes at high pressure.
4. Release the pressure naturally. for 10 minutes, then switch the pressure release valve to Venting to allow any remaining steam out.
5. Spoon the ribs and sauce over cauliflower rice.

Pork Ribs and Pearl Onions Under Pressure

(Prep + Cook Time: 35 minutes / Servings: 4)

Ingredients:

- 1 pound Pork Ribs
- 2 Tbsp. olive oil
- 1 ¼ cups Pearl Onions
- 1 ½ cups Tomato Sauce from deseeded / peeled tomatoes
- 1 tbsp minced Garlic
- ½ tsp Pepper
- ¾ tsp Salt
- 1 ½ cups Water

Directions:

1. Cut the ribs into individual pieces, then season with salt and pepper.
2. Set your Instant Pot to SAUTÉ, heat the oil and brown the ribs in it. Add the onion and garlic and cook for 2 minutes more.
3. Pour the tomato sauce and water into the Instant Pot.
4. Lock the lid and set the Pressure Release to Sealing. Select MEAT/STEW and cook for 30 minutes at high pressure.
5. Release the pressure naturally for 10 minutes. Serve hot.

Barbecue Pork Butt

(Prep + Cook Time: 55 minutes / Servings: 4)

Ingredients:

- 2 ¼ pounds Pork Butt
- ¼ tsp Garlic Powder
- ¼ tsp Pepper
- 1 cup Barbecue Sauce
- ¼ tsp Cumin Powder
- ½ tsp Onion Powder
- 1 ½ cup Beef Broth

Directions:

1. Coat your Instant Pot with cooking oil and set it to SAUTÉ.
2. Combine the barbecue sauce and all of the spices. Brush this mixture over the pork. Place the pork in the cooker and sear on all sides.
3. Pour the beef broth around the meat.
4. Close the lid and cook for 40 minutes on MEAT/STEW at high pressure. When the cooking cycle ends, allow pressure to release naturally for 10 minutes.
5. Serve the pork with coleslaw, along with extra barbecue sauce on the side.

Pork Chops and Mushrooms in a Tomato Sauce

(Prep + Cook Time: 35minutes / Servings: 4)

Ingredients:

- 4 large Bone-In Pork Chops
- 1 cup Tomato Sauce from deseeded / peeled tomatoes
- 1 ½ cups sliced White Button Mushrooms
- 1 Onion, chopped
- 1 tsp minced Garlic
- ½ cup Water
- 1 tbsp Oil
- Salt and Pepper, to taste

Directions:

1. Heat the oil in your Instant Pot on SAUTÉ. Add garlic and onion and cook for 2 minutes.
2. Add pork and cook until browned on all sides, about 4-5 minutes per side. Stir in the remaining ingredients and close the lid.
3. Cook on MEAT/STEW for 20 minutes at high pressure. Allow the pressure to release naturally for 10 minutes.
4. Serve the pork chops with mushrooms on top.

Pork with Rutabaga and Granny Smith Apples

(Prep + Cook Time: 40 minutes / Servings: 4)

Ingredients:

- 1 pound Pork Loin, cut into cubes
- 1 Onion, diced
- 2 Rutabagas, peeled and diced
- 1 cup Chicken Broth
- ½ cup White Wine
- 2 Granny Smith Apples, peeled and diced
- ½ cup sliced Leeks
- 1 tbsp Vegetable Oil
- 1 Celery Stalk, diced
- 2 tbsp dried Parsley
- ¼ tsp Thyme
- ½ tsp Cumin
- ¼ tsp Lemon Zest
- Salt and Pepper, to taste

Directions:

1. Season the pork with salt and pepper. Heat the oil in your Instant Pot on SAUTÉ mode.
2. Add the pork and cook for a few minutes, until browned.
3. Stir in the onions and cook for 2 more minutes.
4. Add in the remaining ingredients, except the apples. Close the lid and cook for 15 minutes on MEAT/STEW at high pressure.
5. When the cooking cycle ends, allow pressure to release naturally for 10 minutes.
6. Stir in the apples, close the lid again, and cook on MEAT/STEW for another 5 minutes. Serve hot.

Spicy Ground Pork

(Prep + Cook Time: 55 minutes / Servings: 6)

Ingredients:

- 2 pounds Ground Pork
- 1 Onion, diced
- 5 Garlic Cloves, crushed
- 3 tbsp Ghee Butter
- 1 Serrano Pepper, chopped
- ⅔ cup Beef Broth
- 1 tsp ground Ginger
- 2 tsp ground Coriander
- 1 tsp Salt
- ¾ tsp Cumin
- ¼ tsp Cayenne Pepper
- ½ tsp Turmeric
- ½ tsp Black Pepper
- ¼ cup thinly sliced scallions

Directions:

1. Set your Instant Pot to SAUTÉ and melt the butter in it.
2. Stir in the onions and cook for 3 minutes.
3. Add the spices and garlic and cook for 2 more minutes.
4. Then, add the pork and cook until browned.
5. Finally, pour the beef broth and add the serrano pepper.
6. Close the lid and cook for 30 minutes on MEAT/STEW at high pressure.
7. When the cooking cycle ends, allow pressure to natural release for 10 minutes.
8. Garnish with the scallions and serve over cauliflower rice or mixed vegetables.

Pork Chops in Merlot

(Prep + Cook Time: 30 minutes / Servings: 4)

Ingredients:

- 4 Pork Chops
- 3 Carrots, chopped
- 1 Tomato, chopped
- 1 Onion, chopped
- 2 Garlic Cloves, minced
- 4 ounces Merlot
- 1 tsp dried Oregano
- 2 tbsp Olive Oil
- 2 tbsp Almond Flour
- 2 tbsp Water
- 2 tbsp Tomato Paste
- 1 Beef Bouillon Cube
- ¼ tsp Pepper
- ¼ tsp Salt
- 1 tbsp chives, thinly sliced (for garnish)

Directions:

1. Set your Instant Pot on SAUTÉ and heat the oil in it.
2. Toss the pork chops with the flour, pepper, and salt.
3. Place in the cooker and cook for a few minutes, until browned on all sides.
4. Add the carrots, garlic, and oregano. Cook for 3 minutes more.
5. Stir in the remaining ingredients and close the lid. Choose MEAT/STEW and cook for 25 minutes at high pressure.
6. Do a natural pressure release for 10 minutes and serve.
7. Transfer the pork chops to a serving platter and garnish with chives.

Beef Cabbage Rolls in a Tomato Sauce

(Prep + Cook Time: 55 minutes / Servings: 5)

Ingredients:

- 10 Cabbage Leaves, blanched
- 1 ½ pounds ground Beef
- 2 cups Cauliflower Rice, cooked
- 1 tbsp minced Garlic
- 15 ounces Tomato Sauce from deseeded / peeled tomatoes
- 1 Onion, chopped
- ½ tsp Cayenne Pepper
- Salt and Pepper, to taste
- Small bunch fresh basil, chopped, to serve

Directions:

1. In a bowl, combine the beef, cauliflower rice, cayenne pepper, garlic, tomato sauce, and onions.
2. Divide this mixture among the cabbage rolls and roll them up. Arrange the rolls in the Instant Pot.
3. Close the lid and cook on MEAT/STEW for 40 minutes at high pressure.
4. When the cooking cycle ends, allow pressure to release naturally for 10 minutes.
5. Scatter with basil leaves and serve 2 per person.

Braised Chili Pork Chops

(Prep + Cook Time: 30 minutes / Servings: 4)

Ingredients:

- 4 Pork Chops
- 1 Onion, chopped
- 2 tbsp Chili Powder
- 1 Garlic Clove, minced
- ½ cup Beer
- 1 tsp Oil
- 1 tblsp chives, thinly sliced (for garnish)

Directions:

1. Heat the oil in your Instant Pot on SAUTÉ.
2. Add onion, garlic, and chili powder and cook for 2 minutes.
3. Add the pork chops and cook until browned on all sides.
4. Stir in the beer. Season with salt and pepper.
5. Close the lid and cook on MANUAL for 20 minutes at high pressure.
6. Release the pressure naturally for 10 minutes and serve.
7. Place chops on a platter and garnish with the chives.

Beef Ribs with Button Mushrooms

(Prep + Cook Time: 30 minutes / Servings: 4)

Ingredients:

- 2 pounds Beef Ribs
- 2 cups quartered White Button Mushrooms
- 1 Onion, chopped
- ¼ cup Ketchup homemade from deseeded / peeled tomatoes.
- 2 ½ cups Veggie Stock
- ¼ cup Olive Oil
- 1 tsp minced Garlic
- Salt and Pepper, to taste

Directions:

1. Heat the oil in your Instant Pot on SAUTÉ. Season the ribs with salt and pepper and brown them on all sides. Set aside.
2. Add the onion, garlic, and mushrooms and cook for 3-4 minutes, stirring well.
3. Add the ribs back to the cooker and stir in the remaining ingredients. Close the lid and cook for 35 minutes on MEAT/STEW at high pressure.
4. Allow the pressure to release naturally for 10 minutes.
5. Carefully open the lid and taste, adding more salt and pepper if necessary.
6. Transfer the ribs to a platter drizzled with the mushroom sauce.

Beef Medley with Blue Cheese Roquefort and Cabbage

(Prep + Cook Time: 50 minutes / Servings: 6)

Ingredients:

- 1 pound Sirloin Steak, cut into cubes
- 6 ounces Goat brie
- ½ Cabbage, diced
- 1 cup chopped Parsnip
- ½ cup Beef Broth
- 1 Onion, diced
- 1 tsp minced Garlic
- Salt and Pepper, to taste

Directions:

1. Coat the Instant Pot with cooking spray and brown the steak on SAUTÉ.
2. Add the remaining ingredients, except the cheese.
3. Close the lid and cook for 40 minutes on MEAT/STEW.
4. Release the pressure naturally. Top with the cheese and serve.

Worcestershire Beef Brisket

(Prep + Cook Time: 60 minutes / Servings: 4)

Ingredients:

- 1 ½ pounds Beef Brisket
- 1 tbsp Worcestershire Sauce
- 1 tsp Onion Powder
- 1 tbsp Ketchup
- 1 tsp minced Garlic
- 2 cups Beef Stock
- 1 tbsp Stevia Brown Sugar
- 2 tbsp Apple Cider Vinegar
- 1 tsp Cayenne Pepper
- ¼ tsp Pepper
- ½ tsp Salt

Directions:

1. Place the beef in your Instant Pot. Whisk together the remaining ingredients in a bowl.
2. Pour the mixture over the beef, close the lid and select MANUAL.
3. Cook for 40 minutes at high pressure. Release the pressure naturally for 10 minutes.
4. Slice brisket 1-inch thick. Drizzle the liquid over brisket to serve.

Basil and Thyme Pot Roast

(Prep + Cook Time: 55 minutes / Servings: 6)

Ingredients:

- 2 pounds Beef Roast, cubed
- 2 Yams, chopped
- 4 Garlic Cloves, minced
- 1 Red Onion, chopped
- 1 ½ cups Bone Broth

- ½ tbsp dried Basil
- 2 tsp dried Thyme
- 1 cup Tomato Paste
- 2 tsp Oil
- Salt and Pepper, to taste

Directions:

1. Season the meat with salt and pepper. Heat the oil in the cooker on SAUTÉ. Add the meat and cook until browned. Stir in the remaining ingredients.
2. Close the lid and cook for 40 minutes on MEAT/STEW at high pressure.
3. Wait 5 minutes and do a quick pressure release. Serve immediately.

Sweet Balsamic Beef

(Prep + Cook Time: 55 minutes / Servings: 8)

Ingredients:

- 3 pounds Chuck Steak, sliced
- 5 dropd Stevia liquid
- ½ cup Balsamic Vinegar
- 1 cup Bone Broth
- 1 tsp minced Garlic
- 1 tsp Salt
- 2 tbsp Olive Oil
- 1 tsp ground Ginger

Directions:

1. Heat the oil in your Instant Pot on SAUTÉ.
2. Season the beef with salt and ginger. Brown on all sides in the pot.
3. Stir well in the remaining ingredients.
4. Close the lid and cook for 45 minutes on MEAT/STEW at high pressure.
5. Let the pressure to release naturally, for 10 minutes, and serve warm.

Beef in a Creamy Sour Sauce

(Prep + Cook Time: 35 minutes / Servings: 6)

Ingredients:

- 1 ½ pounds Beef Roast, cubed
- 1 cup diced Onions
- 1 can Cream of Mushroom Soup
- 1 ½ cups Organic Sour Cream
- ½ tbsp Cumin
- 1 tbsp minced Garlic
- 1 tbsp Ghee Butter
- ½ tsp Chili Powder
- Salt and Pepper, to taste
- ½ tbsp fresh Coriander, chopped to garnish

Directions:

1. Melt the butter in your Instant Pot on SAUTÉ and cook the onions until soft. Add garlic and cook for one more minute. Add the beef and cook until browned.
2. Combine the remaining ingredients in a bowl and pour this mixture over the beef. Close the lid and cook for 20 minutes on MEAT/STEW at higth pressure.
3. Allow the pressure to release naturally for 10 minutes. Garnish with fresh coriander and serve.

Ground Beef, Leek, and Sauerkraut

(Prep + Cook Time: 50 minutes / Servings: 6)

Ingredients:

- 1 ½ pounds Ground Beef
- 10 ounces canned Tomato Soup
- 3 cups Sauerkraut
- 1 cup sliced Leeks
- 1 tbsp Ghee Butter

- 1 tsp Mustard Powder
- Salt and Pepper, to taste
- chopped fresh Italian parsley to garnis

Directions:

1. Melt the butter in the Instant Pot on SAUTÉ.
2. Place the leeks and cook them for a few minutes, until tender.
3. Add beef and cook until browned. Stir in the sauerkraut and mustard powder and season with salt and pepper.
4. Close the lid and cook for 15 minutes on MANUAL mode at higth pressure.
5. Allow the pressure to release naturally for 10 minutes. Release any remaining steam. Garnish with parsley to serve.

Corned Beef in a Celery Sauce

(Prep + Cook Time: 50 minutes / Servings: 4-6)

Ingredients:

- 1 ½ pounds Corned Beef Brisket
- 1 ½ cups Cream of Celery Soup
- 1 tsp minced Garlic
- 1 Onion, diced
- 2 tsp Oil
- Salt and Pepper, to taste
- Chopped fresh parsley (optional)

Directions:

1. Season the beef with salt and pepper. Heat the oil in the Instant Pot on SAUTÉ.
2. Stir in the onions and cook for 2 minutes or untin translucent. Add garlic and cook for one more minute.
3. Add beef and sear on all sides. Pour the celery soup over.
4. Close the lid and cook for 40 minutes on MEAT/STEW at high pressure.

5. Allow the pressure to release naturally for 10 minutes. Release any remaining steam.
6. Serve with vegetables and sauce. Garnish with parsley.

Beef Sausage and Red Cabbage Casserole

(Prep + Cook Time: 30 minutes / Servings: 4)

Ingredients:

- 1 pound Beef Sausage, crumbled
- 1 pound Red Cabbage, shredded
- 1 ½ cups Tomato Puree
- 1 cup Cauliflower Rice
- 1 tbsp Cider Vinegar
- ½ tsp Fennel Seeds
- ⅓ cup chopped Scallions
- Salt and Pepper, to taste

Directions:

1. Season the cabbage with the fennel in a bowl. Place half of this mixture in the Instant Pot. Combine the sausage, cauliflower rice, and scallions in another bowl.
2. Place half of this mixture over the cabbage. Repeat the layers. Whisk together the vinegar, tomato puree, salt and pepper.
3. Pour this mixture over the sausage. Close the lid and cook on MEAT/STEW for 15 minutes at high pressure. Allow the pressure to release naturally.
4. Spoon the cabbage onto a heated platter, top it with the sausage and serve.

Drunken Beef and Mushrooms

(Prep + Cook Time: 60 minutes / Servings: 6)

Ingredients:

- 2 pounds Beef Roast
- 1 pound White Button Mushrooms, quartered
- 2 tbsp Tomato Paste
- 1 Onion, chopped
- 1 tsp minced Garlic
- 1 cup Red Wine
- 1 cup Beef Broth
- 1 deseeded / peeled Tomato,
- 1 tbsp Olive Oil
- ¼ tsp Pepper
- ¼ tsp Salt
- 2 medium scallions (green parts only), thinly sliced

Directions:

1. Heat the oil in your Instant Pot on SAUTÉ. Season the beef with salt and pepper.
2. Sauté the onion for 2 minutes. Add beef and sear on all sides. Whisk together the remaining ingredients in a bowl.
3. Pour over the meat. Close the lid and cook for 40 minutes on MEAT/STEW.
4. Release the pressure naturally for about 10 minutes.
5. Top with the scallions, and serve warm.

Dark Beer and Dijon Braised Steak

(Prep + Cook Time: 40 minutes / Servings: 4)

Ingredients:

- 4 Beef Steaks
- 12 ounces Dark Beer
- 2 tbsp Dijon Mustard
- 1 tbsp Tomato Paste
- 1 Onion, chopped
- 1 tsp Paprika

- 2 tbsp Flour
- 1 cup Beef Broth
- Salt and Pepper, to taste
- Fresh basil, snipped to garnish

Directions:

1. Brush the meat with the mustard and sprinkle with paprika, salt, and pepper.
2. Coat the Instant Pot with cooking spray and sear the steak on SAUTÉ. Transfer the steaks to a plate. Pour ¼ cup beer and scrape the bottom of the cooker.
3. Whisk in the tomato paste and flour. Gradually stir in the remaining ingredients.
4. Return the steaks to the cooker and close the lid.
5. Cook for 15 minutes on MANUAL at high pressure.
6. Release the pressure naturally.
7. Transfer the steaks to a plate. Garnish with the fresh basil.

Tender Onion Beef Roast

(Prep + Cook Time: 55 minutes / Servings: 8)

Ingredients:

- 3 pounds Beef Roast
- 2 Large Sweet Onions, sliced
- 1 envelope Onion Mix
- 1 cup Beef Broth
- 1 cup Tomato Juice, from deseeded / peeled tomatoes
- 1 tsp minced Garlic
- 1 tbsp Worcestershire Sauce
- 1 tbsp Olive Oil
- 1 Bay Leaf
- Salt and Pepper, to taste

Directions:

1. Heat the oil in your Instant Pot on SAUTÉ.
2. Season the beef with salt and pepper and sear it on all sides. Transfer to a plate.
3. Stir in the onions and cook for 3 minutes. Add garlic and cook for 1 more minutes. Then, add the beef and stir in the remaining ingredients.
4. Close the lid and cook for 40 minutes on MANUAL mode. Release the pressure naturally for about 10 minutes.
5. Remove and discard the bay leaf. Transfer beef to a large serving platter. Serve with vegetables.

Mexican Brisket

(Prep + Cook Time: 55 minutes / Servings: 6)

Ingredients:

- 2 ½ pounds Beef Brisket
- 1 tbsp Chili Powder
- 1 tbsp Tomato Paste
- ½ cup Salsa
- ½ cup Beef Broth
- 1 tbsp Ghee Butter
- 1 Spanish Onion, sliced
- 2 Garlic Cloves, minced

Directions:

1. Season the beef with chili powder.
2. Coat the Instant Pot with cooking spray and SAUTÉ the beef until browned on all sides. Add onion and cook for 2 more minutes.
3. Stir in the remaining ingredients.
4. Close the lid and press MEAT/STEW.
5. Cook on high for 35 minutes. Once ready, perform a quick pressure release and serve hot.

Spicy Shredded Beef

(Prep + Cook Time: 3 hours / Servings: 8)

Ingredients:

- 3 pounds Beef Roast
- ½ cup Ketchup
- ½ cup Red Wine
- 1 cup Water
- 2 tsp coconut aminos
- 1 tbsp Stevia Brown Sugar
- 1 tbsp Balsamic Vinegar
- 2 tbsp minced Onions
- 2 tsp Mustard Powder
- 1 tsp Chili Powder
- 1 tsp minced Garlic
- ¼ tsp Nutmeg
- ½ tsp Cinnamon
- 1 tsp Pepper
- ¼ tsp Salt
- ¼ tsp Ginger

Directions:

1. Place the beef in your Instant Pot. Whisk together the remaining ingredients in a bowl. Pour this mixture over the beef.
2. Close the lid and cook for 3 hours on SLOW COOK mode.
3. Once ready, let the pressure to release naturally, for 20 minutes, then set steam vent to Venting to quick-release remaining pressure.
4. Serve hot with mashed cauliflower.

Bourbon and Apricot Meatloaf

(Prep + Cook Time: 30 minutes / Servings: 4)

Ingredients:

1 ½ cups Water

Meatloaf:

- 1 pound ground Beef
- 1 Egg White
- ⅔ cup Pork Rinds
- 2 tbsp Ketchup
- ⅔ cup diced Onion
- ½ tsp Basil
- 1 tsp minced Garlic

Glaze:

- 1 cup Apricot Jam
- ½ cup Bourbon
- ½ cup Barbecue Sauce
- ¼ cup Honey
- ¼ cup Water
- 1 tbsp Hot Sauce

Directions:

1. Combine all of the meatloaf ingredients in a bowl. Shape into a meatloaf and place on a greased pan that can fit in your Instant Pot.
2. Whisk the glaze ingredients in a bowl. Brush this mixture over the meatloaf. Set your cooker to MEAT/STEW and pour the water inside.
3. Place the baking dish in the Instant Pot and close the lid. Cook for 50 minutes at high pressure.
4. Allow the pressure to release naturally for 10 minutes, then set steam vent to Venting to quick-release remaining pressure.

Teriyaki and Peach Pulled Beef

(Prep + Cook Time: 5 hours / Servings: 10)

Ingredients:

- 4 pounds Beef Roast
- ½ cup Teriyaki Sauce
- ½ cup Peach Preserves
- ½ cup Ketchup
- ¼ cup Apple Cider Vinegar
- ¼ cup Stevia Brown Sugar
- 1 tsp Dijon Mustard
- 1 ½ cups Water
- 1 Onion, sliced
- 2 bay leaves
- ½ tsp Pepper
- Pinch of Salt

Directions:

1. Cut the meat in 4 equal pieces and stir in the remaining ingredients.
2. Cover and let marinate for 50-60 minutes. Place the beef along with the marinade in the Instant Pot.
3. Close the lid and cook on SLOW COOK mode for 4 hours.
4. Remove the bay leaves. tently shred the beef with two forks.
5. Top with the remaining half of the parsley. Serve over cauliflower rice.

Marinated Flank Steak

(Prep + Cook Time: 80 minutes / Servings: 4)

Ingredients:

- 2 pounds grass-fed Flank Steak
- ½ cup Beef Broth
- 1 Onion, diced

Marinade:

- 2 tbsp Fish Sauce
- ½ tsp Cajun Seasoning
- 2 tsp minced Garlic
- ½ cup coconut aminos
- 1 tbsp Sesame Oil

Directions:

1. Combine the marinade ingredients in a bowl. Add the beef and let marinate for 30 minutes. Coat the pot with cooking spray.
2. Stir in the onions and cook until soft on SAUTÉ. Add the beef along with the marinade.
3. Whisk in the broth and starch. Close the lid and cook for 40 minutes MEAT/STEW at high pressure. Qucik release the pressure and serve.

Coconut Beef with Plantains

(Prep + Cook Time: 50 minutes / Servings: 4)

Ingredients:

- 1 ¾ pound Beef Roast, cubed
- 1 cup Coconut Milk
- 2 Onions, sliced
- 1 Plantain, chopped
- 1 tbsp Coconut Oil
- 1 tsp ground Ginger
- 1 tsp Garlic Powder
- ½ tsp Turmeric

Directions:

1. Season the beef with all of the spices. Melt the coconut oil in your Instant Pot. Add the beef and cook until brown on SAUTÉ.
2. Add onions and cook for 3 more minutes.
3. Pour the coconut milk over and close the lid. Cook for 30 minutes on MANUAL at high pressure. Once ready, do a quick pressure release.
4. Stir in the plantain. Cook for another 5-7 minutes. Serve hot.

Herbed Beef Cubes

(Prep + Cook Time: 35 minutes / Servings: 6)

Ingredients:

- 3 pounds Beef Roast, cut into cubes
- 2 tsp Thyme
- 2 tsp Oregano
- 2 tsp Parsley
- 2 tsp Rosemary
- 2 minced Garlic Cloves
- 2 tbsp Olive Oil
- 3 tbsp Flour
- ½ tsp salt
- ¼ tsp Pepper
- 1 ½ cups Beef Broth

Directions:

1. Heat the oil in your Instant Pot on SAUTÉ.
2. Season the beef with the salt and pepper and toss with flour. Cook until browned on all sides.
3. Stir in the remaining ingredients and close the lid.
4. Cook for 30 minutes on MEAT/STEW mode at high pressure.
5. Press CANCEL and release the pressure naturally for 10 minutes.
6. Release any remaining steam and serve immediately.

Simple Cheesy Meatballs

(Prep + Cook Time: 30 minutes / Servings: 4)

Ingredients:

- 1 pound ground Beef
- ½ cup diced Onion
- 1 Egg
- ½ tsp Garlic Powder
- ½ cup crumbled Sheep Feta Cheese
- 1 tbsp mixed dried Herbs
- ½ cup Pork Rinds
- ¼ tsp Pepper
- 1 cup canned Cream of Mushroom Soup
- ¼ cup Water
- ½ cup grated Sheep Cheese

Directions:

1. In a bowl, combine the first 8 ingredients. Shape into meatballs.
2. Coat the Instant Pot with cooking spray on SAUTÉ.
3. Add the meatballs and brown on all sides.
4. Pour the water and soup over, close the lid and cook for 15 minutes on MANUAL mode at high pressure.
5. Perform a quick release, open the lid, and stir in the sheep cheese.
6. Cook for additional 3 minutes. Serve immediately.

Poultry

Chicken in Beer Sauce

(Prep + Cook Time: 40 minutes / Servings: 4)

Ingredients:

- 1 ½ pounds Chicken Breasts
- 10 ounces Beer
- 1 cup chopped Green Onions
- 1 ¼ cup Goat yogurt
- ⅓ cup Arrowroot
- ½ tsp Sage
- 2 tsp dried Thyme
- 2 tsp dried Rosemary
- 2 tbsp Olive Oil

Directions:

7. Heat the oil in your Instant Pot on SAUTÉ.
8. Stir in the onions and cook them for 2 minutes or until transclucent.
9. Coat the chicken with the arrowroot.
10. Add the chicken to the Instant Pot and cook until browned on all sides.
11. Pour the beer over and bring the mixture to a boil.
12. Stir in the herbs and cook on MANUAL for 30 minutes at high pressure.
13. When the cooking cycle ends, allow pressure to release naturally, for 10 minutes.
14. Stir in the yogurt before serving.

Balsamic Chicken Thighs with Mango

(Prep + Cook Time: 30 minutes / Servings: 6)

Ingredients:

- 6 large Chicken Thighs
- ½ cup chopped Sweet Onions
- 2 Mangos, sliced
- 2 tbsp Balsamic Vinegar
- 3 tsp Ghee Butter
- 1 cup Chicken Broth
- 1 tsp Cayenne Pepper
- Salt and Pepper, to taste

Directions:

1. Melt the ghee in your Instant Pot on SAUTÉ.
2. Add the chicken thighs and sprinkle with the spices.
3. Brown on all sides, for about 5 minutes per side.
4. Stir in the remaining ingredients, except for the mango.
5. Close the lid and press MANUAL.
6. Cook for 20 minutes at high pressure.
7. Once the cooking cycle is over, release the pressure naturally for 10 minutes.
8. Serve the chicken thighs topped with sliced mango.

Lectin Free Coconut Milk Chicken

(Prep + Cook Time: 25 minutes / Servings: 6)

Ingredients:

- 3 pounds Chicken Breasts, boneless and skinless
- 2 cans of Coconut Milk
- 12 ounces canned Tomato Paste
- 1 ½ Onions, chopped
- 1 tbsp Ghee Butter
- 2 tsp Paprika
- 1 ½ tsp Cayenne Powder
- 1 tsp Garlic Powder
- Salt and Pepper, to taste

Directions:

1. Melt the butter in your Instant Pot on SAUTÉ.
2. Add the onions and spices, and sauté for 2 minutes. Then, add the coconut milk and chicken.
3. Close the lid and set valve to Sealing. Select MANUAL and cook for 12 minutes at high pressure.
4. When the cooking cycle ends, allow pressure to release naturally for 10 minutes. Serve the chicken with the cooking liquid.

Sweet and Gingery Whole Chicken

(Prep + Cook Time: 60 minutes / Servings: 6)

Ingredients:

- 1 medium Whole Chicken
- 1 Green Onion, minced
- 2 tbsp Stevia
- 1 tbsp grated Ginger
- 2 tsp coconut aminos
- ¼ cup White Wine
- ½ cup Chicken Broth

- 1 ½ tbsp Olive Oil
- Salt and Pepper, to taste
- ¼ tsp Pepper

Directions:

1. Heat the olive oil in your Instant Pot on SAUTÉ.
2. Season the chicken with the stevia and some salt and pepper; brown on all sides.
3. Whisk together the wine, broth, coconut aminos in the cooker. Add the chicken and seal the lid.
4. Press MANUAL and cook for 35 minutes at high pressure. Release the pressure naturally for 10 minutes. Taste for seasoning and serve.

Habanero Turkey Breasts

(Prep + Cook Time: 30 minutes / Servings: 6)

Ingredients:

- 2 pounds Turkey Breasts
- 6 tbsp Habanero Sauce
- ½ cup Tomato Puree
- 1 ½ cups Water
- ½ tsp Cumin
- 1 tsp Smoked Paprika
- Salt and Pepper, to taste

Directions:

1. Pour the water in your Instant Pot and place a steamer basket on top.
2. Add the turkey and secure the lid. Select MANUAL and cook for 15 minutes at high pressure.
3. When the cooking cycle ends, allow pressure to release naturally for 10 minutes. Open the lid and discard the cooking liquid.
4. Shred the turkey within the pot and add the remaining ingredients.
5. Cook on SAUTÉ with the lid off for a few minutes, or until thickened.

Cranberry Turkey Wings

(Prep + Cook Time: 40 minutes / Servings: 4)

Ingredients:

- 1 pound Turkey Wings
- 1 stick of Ghee Butter
- 1 cup Cranberries
- 2 Onions, sliced
- 2 cups Veggie Stock
- ½ tsp Cayenne Pepper
- Salt and Black Pepper, to taste

Directions:

1. Melt the butter in the Instant Pot on SAUTÉ. Season the turkey wings with salt, black and cayenne pepper.
2. Once the butter is melted, add the turkey chicken and cook until browned, about 4-5 minutes. Remove the turkey.
3. Stir in the onions and cook for 3 minutes, or until is translucent. Pour in the stock and cranberries. Season with salt and pepper, and give it a good stir.
4. Close the lid and set valve to Sealing. Press MANUAL and cook for 25 minutes at high pressure.
5. Once ready, release the pressure naturally for 10 minutes. Serve the turkey with the cooking liquid.

Curry and Coconut Milk Chicken

(Prep + Cook Time: 25 minutes / Servings: 4)

Ingredients:

- 1 pound boneless and skinless Chicken Breasts
- ½ cup Coconut Milk
- ½ tsp Turmeric
- 2 tsp Curry Paste
- 1 tsp Stevia
- Salt and Pepper, to taste

Directions:

1. Chop the chicken into cubes and place them in the Instant Pot. Season with salt and pepper. Stir in the remaining ingredients.
2. Close the lid and set valve to Sealing. Seletct MANUAL, and cook for 25 minutes at high pressure.
3. Allow the pressure to release naturally for at least 10 minutes. Carefully open the lid and taste, add some salt and pepper if necessary.
4. Serve the chicken with the cooking liquid.

Mustard and Lime Goose

(Prep + Cook Time: 30 minutes / Servings: 4)

Ingredients:

- 1 pound skinless and boneless Goose Meat, cut into cubes
- ½ cup White Wine
- 1 tbsp Dijon Mustard
- 1 tbsp minced Garlic
- 2 tbsp Oil
- Juice from 1 Lime
- ¼ tsp Thyme
- ¼ tsp Oregano
- Salt and Pepper, to taste
- ¼ cup Chicken Broth

Directions:

1. Heat the oil in your Instant Pot on SAUTÉ. Add the goose meat and brown for 5 minutes.
2. Add the remaining ingredients and stir to coat well. Seal the lid and cook for 10 minutes on MAUAL at high pressure.
3. Release the pressure naturally for 10 minutes. Transfer the goose to a plate.
4. On Sauté mode, cook the sauce with the lid off for a few minutes, until thickened. Add the meat and stir to coat well. Serve hot.

Turkey Meatloaf

(Prep + Cook Time: 30 minutes / Servings: 4)

Ingredients:

- 1 ½ pounds ground Turkey
- 1 Onion, diced
- 1 Celery Stalk, diced
- ½ cup pork rinds
- 1 Egg
- 3 tbsp Ketchup
- 1 tsp minced Garlic
- ½ tsp Thyme
- ¼ tsp Oregano
- ¼ tsp Salt
- ¼ tsp Pepper
- 1 tsp Worcestershire Sauce
- 1 ½ cup Water

Directions:

1. Pour the water in your Instant Pot pressure cooker.
2. Combine all of the remaining ingredients in a large bowl.
3. Grease a pan with cooking spray and press the mixture in it. Lower the trivet and place the pan inside your Instant Pot.
4. Close the lid and cook on MANUAL for 15 minutes at high pressure.
5. Release the pressure naturally for 10 minutes. Let rest 10 minutes before slicing. Serve with steamed vegetables.

Balsamic Chicken

(Prep + Cook Time: 30 minutes / Servings: 4)

Ingredients:

- 4 Chicken Breasts, boneless and skinless
- 2 tbsp Balsamic Vinegar

- 1 cup Water
- 1 tsp Thyme
- ½ tsp Rosemary
- 1 Garlic Clove, minced
- Pinch of Black Pepper

Directions:

1. Rub the chicken with pepper, rosemary, thyme, and garlic.
2. Place it in the Instant Pot.
3. In a bowl, whisk together the water and vinegar. Pour the mixture over the chicken.
4. Press MANUAL and cook for 20 minutes at high pressure. Allow the pressure to release naturally for 10 minutes.

Simple Garlicky Goose

(Prep + Cook Time: 70 minutes / Servings: 5)

Ingredients:

- ½ medium Goose, cut into pieces
- 1 Onion, chopped
- 12 ounces canned Mushroom Soup
- 2 tsp minced Garlic
- 3 ½ cups Water
- Salt and Pepper, to taste
- 1 tablespoon thinly sliced fresh chives to garnish

Directions:

1. Place the water, goose, onion, and garlic in your Instant Pot.
2. Close the lid and cook on MEAT/STEW for an hour at high pressure.
3. Stir in the mushroom soup and season with salt and pepper.
4. Cook for 5 minutes with the lid off. Garnish with chives to serve.

Thyme and Lemon Drumsticks

(Prep + Cook Time: 35 minutes / Servings: 4)

Ingredients:

- 4 Chicken Drumsticks
- 1 Onion, sliced
- 2 tsp dried Thyme
- 1 tsp Lemon Zest
- 2 tbsp Lemon Juice
- 1 tbsp Olive Oil
- Salt and Pepper, to taste

Directions:

1. Heat the olive oil in your Instant Pot on SAUTÉ.
2. Add the drumsticks and brown for 5 minutes. Stir in the remaining ingredients.
3. Lock pressure cooker lid in place and set steam vent handle to Sealing.
4. Press MANUAL and cook for 15 minutes at high pressure. Release the pressure naturally for 10 minutes then release, the steam.

Smoked Paprika Chicken Legs

(Prep + Cook Time: 30 minutes / Servings: 4)

Ingredients:

- 4 Chicken Legs (about 8-ounce each)
- 1 Onion, chopped
- 1 reduced-lectin Tomato, chopped
- ½ cup Organic sour cream
- ½ cup Chicken Broth
- 1 tbsp Olive Oil
- 2 tsp Smoked Paprika
- ½ tsp Garlic Powder
- Salt and Pepper to taste

Directions:

1. Season the chicken with salt, pepper, garlic powder, and smoked paprika.
2. Heat the oil in your Instant Pot on SAUTÉ and brown the chicken legs on all sides. Stir in the remaining ingredients and seal the lid.
3. Set MANUAL and cook for 15 minutes at high pressure. Release the pressure naturally. This might take 10 minutes.
4. Garnish with desired toppings to serve.

Bacon and Cheese Shredded Chicken

(Prep + Cook Time: 40 minutes / Servings: 4)

Ingredients:

- 4 Chicken Breasts
- 8 ounces Organic cream cheese
- 2 cups shredded Goat cheese
- ¼ cup chopped Scallion
- 4 ounces chopped Bacon
- 1 cup Mayonnaise (avocado and oil based)
- ½ cup Chicken Broth
- 2 tsp Ranch Seasoning

Directions:

1. Press SAUTÉ on your pressure cooker. Add the bacon and cook until crispy, about 3-4 minutes. Transfer the bacon to a plate.
2. Add chicken, broth, cream cheese, and ranch dressing.
3. Seal the lid, press MANUAL and cook for 15 minutes at high pressure.
4. Release the pressure naturally for 10 minutes. Shred the chicken with two forks inside the Instant Pot.
5. Stir in the remaining ingredients and cook for 2 more minutes.
6. Allow the pressure to release naturally, for 10 minutes. Serve topped with the crispy bacon.

Mexican Turkey Breasts

(Prep + Cook Time: 35 minutes / Servings: 4)

Ingredients:

- 24 ounces Turkey Breasts, frozen
- 1 cup shredded Buffalo mozzarella (made from buffalo milk)
- 1 cup mild Salsa
- 1 cup Tomato Sauce from deseeded / peeled tomatoes.
- 3 tbsp Lime Juice
- Salt and Pepper, to taste

Directions:

1. Place the tomato sauce, salsa, lime juice, and turkey in your Instant Pot.
2. Close the lid nd seal it. Select MANUAL and cook for 15 minutes. Do a natural pressure release for 10 minutes.
3. Shred the turkey inside the Instant Pot and stir in the cheese. Cook for another minute on MANUAL. Serve immediately

Garlic and Thyme Chicken

(Prep + Cook Time: 40 minutes / Servings: 4-6)

Ingredients:

- 3 ½ pound Whole Chicken
- 1 tbsp dried Thyme
- Juice from 1 Lemon
- 3 Garlic Cloves
- 2 cups Chicken Broth
- ½ tsp Pepper
- ½ tsp Salt
- 1 tbsp Olive Oil

Directions:

1. Season the chicken with salt, pepper, and thyme.
2. Heat the olive oil in your Instant Pot on SAUTÉ and brown the chicken with the breast-side down.
3. Add garlic and cook for 30 more seconds.
4. Pour the broth and lemon juice around (not over!) the chicken.
5. Close the lid nd seal it. Select MANUAL and cook for 25 minutes at high pressure.
6. Release the pressure naturally for 10 minutes.
7. Transfer the chicken to a cutting board to rest for 5 minutes before carving.

Basil and Oregano Duck Breasts

(Prep + Cook Time: 30 minutes / Servings: 4)

Ingredients:

- 18 ounces Duck Breasts
- 1 tsp dried Oregano
- 1 tsp dried Basil
- 1 tsp Garlic Powder
- 1 ¼ cups Chicken Broth
- 1 tbsp Coconut Oil
- Salt and Pepper, to taste

Directions:

1. Season the duck breasts with the herbs and spices.
2. Melt the coconut oil in your Instant Pot on SAUTÉ.
3. Add the duck and cook until browned, about 5 minutes.
4. Pour the chicken broth over, select MANUAL and close the lid.
5. Cook for 15 minutes at high pressure.
6. Allow the pressure to release naturally, for 10 minutes, and serve.

Vegetable and Side Dishes

Cauliflower and Egg Salad

(Prep + Cook Time: 5 minutes / Servings: 4)

Ingredients:

- 2 ½ cups Cauliflower Florets
- 2 Hardboiled Eggs, sliced
- ¾ cup Water

Dressing:

- 1 ½ tbsp Mayonnaise (avocado and oil based)
- 1 ½ tbsp Sheep Cheese
- 4 tbsp Olive Oil
- 1 Garlic Clove, minced
- 1 canned Anchovy, chopped
- ¼ tsp Mustard
- ¾ tbsp Lemon Juice
- Salt and Pepper, to taste

Directions:

1. Place the cauliflower and water in your Instant Pot.
2. Cook for 2 minutes on MANUAL. Once ready, do a quick pressure release.
3. Drain and transfer to a bowl. Whisk together the dressing ingredients and pour over the cauliflower. Toss to coat. Serve topped with egg slices.

Turmeric Kale with Shallots

(Prep + Cook Time: 20 minutes / Servings: 3)

Ingredients:

- 10 ounces Kale, chopped
- 5 Shallots, chopped

- 1 tsp Turmeric Powder
- 2 tsp Olive Oil
- ½ tsp Coriander Seeds
- ½ tsp Cumin
- Salt and Pepper, to taste

Directions:

1. Pour 1 cup of water in the Instant Pot and place the kale in the steaming basket.
2. Close the lid and cook on MANUAL for 2 minutes.
3. Once ready, do a quick pressure release and transfer to a plate.
4. Discard the water and heat the oil in the pot. Add the spices and shallots and cook until soft.
5. Add in the kale and give it a good stir. Serve immediately

Prosciutto Collards

(Prep + Cook Time: 20 minutes / Servings: 6)

Ingredients:

- 1 ½ cups chopped Collards
- 1 ½ cups diced Scallions
- 2 Garlic Cloves, minced
- 1 pound Prosciutto, diced
- 2 ½ cups Stock
- Salt and Pepper, to taste

Directions:

1. Place the prosciutto and scallions in your Instant Pot and brown them on SAUTÉ. Stir in the remaining ingredients.
2. Close the lid and cook for 10 minutes on MANUAL at high pressure.
3. Once cooking is complete, set steam vent to Venting to quick-release pressure.
4. Serve immediately.

Buttery Golden Beets

(Prep + Cook Time: 30 minutes / Servings: 4)

Ingredients:

- 4 Golden Beets, trimmed
- 2 tbsp Ghee Butter, melted
- ¾ cup Water
- Salt and Pepper, to taste

Directions:

1. Pour the water in your Instant Pot.
2. Place the beets in the steaming basket and cook for 15 minutes on MANUAL. Do a quick pressure release.
3. Let the beets cool for a few minutes, before slicing them.
4. Drizzle with butter and season with salt and pepper.

Broccoli Cheese

(Prep + Cook Time: 5 minutes / Servings: 4)

Ingredients:

- 2 cups Broccoli Florets
- ¼ cup grated Sheep Cheese
- ¾ cup Water
- 2 tbsp Ghee Butter, melted
- Pinch of Salt

Directions:

1. Place the water and broccoli in the Instant Pot.
2. Cook on MANUAL or 2 minutes. Once ready, do a quick pressure release and transfer the florets to a bowl.
3. Add the remaining ingredients and toss well to combine. Serve immediately.

Creamy Goat Cheese Cauliflower

(Prep + Cook Time: 30 minutes / Servings: 5)

Ingredients:

- 1 Cauliflower Head, cut into florets
- 2 tbsp Lemon Juice
- 2 tbsp Olive Oil
- 1 cup Vegetable Broth
- 2 tsp Red Pepper Flakes

Sauce:

- 6 ounces Goat Cheese
- 1 tsp Nutmeg
- ⅓ cup Organic Heavy Cream
- 1 tbsp Olive Oil
- Salt and Pepper, to taste

Directions:

1. Combine the lemon juice and cauliflower in your Instant Pot and cover with water.
2. Lock pressure cooker lid in place and cook for 4 minutes on MANUAL at high pressure. Let pressure release naturally and transfer to a plate.
3. Discard the cooking liquid and heat the oil in the Instant Pot. Add red pepper flakes and cook until fragrant.
4. Add cauliflower and cook for 1 minute uncovered. Return to the bowl.
5. Pulse all of the sauce ingredients in a food processor and pour over the cauliflower.
6. Stir in the basil and season with salt and pepper.

Rutabaga and Scallion Side

(Prep + Cook Time: 10 minutes / Servings: 4)

Ingredients:

- 1 cup minced Scallions
- 2 Rutabagas, cubed
- 1 cup Water
- 3 tsp Orange Juice
- ½ tsp Cayenne Pepper
- ¼ cup Olive Oil
- ¼ tsp Salt

Directions:

1. Combine the water and rutabaga in the Instant Pot and close the lid.
2. Cook on MANUAL for 5 minutes at high pressure. Transfer to a bowl.
3. Release the pressure naturally.
4. Once cooking is complete, allow pressure to release naturally for 10 minutes, then set steam vent to Venting to quick-release remaining pressure.
5. Combine the remaining ingredients and pour over the rutabaga.
6. Toss to combine and serve.

Lime and Mayo Steamed Broccoli

(Prep + Cook Time: 15 minutes / Servings: 6)

Ingredients:

- 1 ½ pounds Broccoli, broken into florets
- ¼ cup Mayonnaise (avocado and oil based)
- ¼ cup Lime Juice
- 1 tsp Cayenne Pepper
- ¼ tsp Garlic Salt
- 1 cup Water

Directions:

1. Combine the water, lime juice, and broccoli in your Instant Pot.
2. Close the lid and cook for 4 minutes on MANUAL at high pressure.
3. Release the pressure naturally for 10 minutes.
4. Carefully remove lid and stir in the remaining ingredients.
5. Serve warm or chilled.

Zesty Onions

(Prep + Cook Time: 15 minutes / Servings: 6)

Ingredients:

- 1 ½ pounds Onions
- 3 tbsp Stevia Brown Sugar
- ¼ cup Wine Vinegar
- 2 tbsp Almond Flour
- 1 cup Water
- 2 Bay Leaves
- 1 tsp Salt
- ½ tsp Pepper

Directions:

1. Combine the onions, bay leaves, and water in the Instant Pot.
2. Close the lid and cook on MANUAL for 4 minutes at high pressure.
3. Release the pressure naturally for about 10 minutes. Transfer to a platter.
4. Get rid of the cooking spray. Whisk together the remaining ingredients in the Instant Pot.
5. Cook for 2 minutes uncovered. Pour the sauce over the onions.

Lemony Brussel Sprouts

(Prep + Cook Time: 30 minutes / Servings: 6)

Ingredients:

- 1 ½ pounds Brussel Sprouts
- 1 ¼ cup Water
- ½ Lemon, sliced
- 1 tbsp Ghee Butter, melted
- Salt and Pepper, to taste

Directions:

1. Combine the lemon slices and Brussel sprouts in the Instant Pot. Add enough water to cover them.
2. Close the lid and cook for 2 minutes on MANUAL at high pressure.
3. Once cooking is complete, allow pressure to release naturally for 10 minutes, then set steam vent to Venting to quick-release remaining pressure.
4. Drizzle with butter and season with salt and pepper.

Balsamic Caper Beets

(Prep + Cook Time: 45 minutes / Servings: 4-6)

Ingredients:

- 4 Beets
- 1 tbsp Olive Oil
- 2 tbsp Capers
- 1 tsp minced Garlic
- 1 tbsp chopped Parsley
- 2 tbsp Balsamic Vinegar
- Salt and Pepper, to taste

Directions:

1. Place the beets in the Instant Pot and cover with water. Cook on MANUAL for 20 minutes.

2. Release the pressure naturally and let the beets cool. Whisk together the remaining ingredients. Slice the beets and combine with the dressing.

Tamari Bok Choy

(Prep + Cook Time: 25 minutes / Servings: 3)

Ingredients:

- 1 Bok Choy Bunch, trimmed
- 2 tbsp Tamari
- 1 tsp minced Garlic
- 2 tbsp Olive Oil
- 1 cup Water
- Salt and Pepper, to taste

Directions:

1. Heat the oil in the Instant Pot and cook the garlic for 1 minute on SAUTÉ.
2. Add the remaining ingredients and close the lid. Select MANUAL and cook for 7 minutes at high pressure.
3. Allow the pressure to release naturally for 10 minutes. Release any remaining steam.

Frascati and Sage Broccoli

(Prep + Cook Time: 15 minutes / Servings: 6)

Ingredients:

- 1 ½ pounds Broccoli, broken into florets
- 1 large Sweet Onion, sliced
- ⅓ cup Frascati
- 2 tsp Sage
- 3 tsp Olive Oil
- 1 tsp Garlic Paste
- Salt and Pepper, to taste

Directions:

1. Heat the oil on SAUTÉ and cook the onions until soft.
2. Add garlic paste and cook until fragrant.
3. Stir in the remaining ingredients. Add some water, if needed.
4. Close the lid and cook for 4 minutes on MANUAL.
5. Allow the pressure to release naturally, for 10 minutes, and serve.

Sweet Caramelized Onions

(Prep + Cook Time: 15 minutes / Servings: 4)

Ingredients:

- 2 large Sweet Onions, peeled
- 1 tbsp Stevia Brown Sugar
- 2 tbsp Ghee Butter
- 1 ½ cup Water

Directions:

1. Place the water and onions in your Instant Pot and cook on SAUTÉ for 5 minutes.
2. Place in ice bath for 2 minutes. Slice and discard the cooking liquid.
3. Melt the butter in the Instant Pot and add the onions and brown sugar.
4. Cook for 5 minutes.

Snacks & Appetizers

Mini Beefy Cabbage Rolls

(Prep + Cook Time: 35 minutes / Servings: 15)

Ingredients:

- 1 Cabbage, leaves separated
- 1 pound ground Beef
- 1 cauliflower rice
- 1 cup Beef Broth
- 3 cups Water
- 2 tbsp Lemon Juice
- 1 Onion, diced
- ⅓ cup Olive Oil
- 1 tsp Fennel Seeds
- Salt and Pepper, to taste

Directions:

1. Place 1 cup of water and the cabbage leaves in the Instant Pot. Close the lid and cook on MANUAL for 2 minutes.
2. Release the pressure naturally. Place in an ice bath to cool.
3. Combine the remaining ingredients except water and broth. Divide this mixture between the cabbage leaves.
4. Roll them up and place in the Instant Pot.
5. Pour the water and broth over. Close the lid and cook for 15 minutes on MEAT/STEW.
6. Allow the pressure to release naturally for 10 minutes and serve immediately.

Buttery Beets

(Prep + Cook Time: 30 minutes / Servings: 4)

Ingredients:

- 1 tbsp Olive Oil
- 1 pound Beets, peeled and sliced
- ½ tsp Garlic Salt
- 4 tbsp Ghee Butter, melted
- 1 tsp dried Basil
- 1 cup Chicken Broth

Directions:

1. Combine the beets and broth in your Instant Pot. Cook on MANUAL for 20 minutes at high pressure.
2. Drain the liquid and sprinkle the beets with olive oil.
3. Cook with the lid off for 5 minutes. Sprinkle with garlic salt and basil and cook for 2 more minutes.
4. Serve drizzled with the melted butter.

Cheese and Polenta Balls

(Prep + Cook Time: 15 minutes / Servings: 6)

Ingredients:

- 2 cups Polenta
- 1 cup chopped Onions
- ½ cup grated Sheep Cheese
- 1 Ghee Butter Stick, melted
- 1 ½ cups Water
- 3 cups Veggie Stock
- ½ tsp Salt
- ¼ tsp Pepper

Directions:

1. Melt 2 tbsp of the butter in your Instant Pot on SAUTÉ.
2. Cook the onions until soft, for a few minutes.
3. Add the water, veggie stock, polenta, pepper, and salt.
4. Close the lid and cook for 10 minutes on MANUAL at high pressure.
5. Once ready, perform a quick pressure release and stir in the cheddar and the rest of the butter.
6. Let cool completely. Make balls out of the mixture and serve chilled.

Sheep Cheese Veggie Appetizer

(Prep + Cook Time: 25 minutes / Servings: 6)

Ingredients:

- 1 cup grated Sheep Cheese
- 1 cup Broccoli Florets
- ¾ tsp Paprika
- ⅓ tsp Cumin Powder
- 1 ½ cups Water
- 2 tbsp Oil
- 1 tsp Salt

Directions:

1. Combine the water, carrots, and broccoli, in your Instant Pot.
2. Close the lid and cook on MANUAL for 15 minutes at high pressure.
3. Once ready, let the pressure release naturally, for 10 minutes
4. While pressure is releasing naturally, drain the veggies and place in a food processor.
5. Add the remaining ingredients and process until smooth.
6. Chill until ready to serve.

Southern Chicken Dip

(Prep + Cook Time: 30 minutes / Servings: 12)

Ingredients:

- 1 pound Chicken Breasts, cut into cubes
- 3 Bacon Slices, chopped
- 1 cup shredded Sheep Cheese
- ½ cup Organic Sour Cream
- ½ cup Salsa
- 1 Onion, diced
- ¼ cup Ketchup
- ½ cup minced Cilantro
- 2 tbsp Olive Oil
- ½ cup Chicken Broth
- 3 Garlic Cloves
- ½ tsp Onion Powder
- 1 tbsp Almond Flour
- ½ tsp Cumin
- ½ tsp Cayenne Pepper
- 1 tsp Chili Powder

Directions:

1. Heat the oil and cook the bacon in your Instant Pot on SAUTÉ.
2. Add onions, cilantro, and garlic. Cook for 3 minutes Stir in the chicken, salsa, broth, and spices.
3. Close the lid and cook for 15 minutes.
4. Release the pressure naturally, for 10 minutes.
5. Whisk in the flour and cook for a few more minutes, until thickened.
6. Transfer to a food processor. Add the cheddar and sour cream.
7. Pulse until smooth.

Minty Grape Leaves

(Prep + Cook Time: 40 minutes / Servings: 12)

Ingredients:

- 16 ounces jarred Grape Leaves
- 1 cup Cauliflower Rice
- ½ cup Mint
- ¼ cup Parsley
- 2 cups Veggie Broth
- Juice from 3 Lemons
- ½ tsp Lemon Zest
- 1 tsp minced Garlic
- 1 tsp Salt
- 4 Scallions, diced

Directions:

1. Coat the Instant Pot with cooking spray.
2. Add scallions, mint, and parsley. Press SAUTÉ and cook for 2 minutes.
3. Stir in the cauliflower rice, broth, zest, and salt. Close the lid and cook on MEAT/STEW for 10 minutes.
4. Release the pressure quickly and transfer to a bowl.
5. Divide the mixture between the grape leaves. Roll them up and arrange in a steamer basket.
6. Drizzle the lemon juice over and cover with foil.
7. Close the lid and cook for 10 more minutes.

Salmon Bites

(Prep + Cook Time: 15 minutes / Servings: 4)

Ingredients:

- 1 can Salmon, flaked
- 1 Spring Onion, minced
- 1 cup Pork Rinds
- ½ cup Organic Cream Cheese
- 1 tbsp chopped Parsley
- ¼ tsp Salt
- ¼ tsp Pepper
- 1 tbsp Ghee Butter
- ½ cup Tomato Sauce, from deseeded / peeled tomatoes
- 1 cup Water

Directions:

1. Combine the first 7 ingredients in a bowl. Make balls out of the mixture.
2. Melt the butter in the Instant Pot on SAUTÉ. Add the balls and cook until golden on all sides.
3. Transfer to a baking dish and pour the tomato sauce over.
4. Pour the water in your Instant Pot and lower the trivet. Place the dish inside and close the lid.
5. Cook for 4 minutes on MANUAL mode.
6. Once ready, release the pressure naturally for about 15 minutes.

Chili Sriracha Eggs

(Prep + Cook Time: 20 minutes / Servings: 6)

Ingredients:

- 6 Eggs
- ½ tsp Chili Powder
- 1 ½ tbsp Organic Sour Cream
- 1 tbsp Mayonnaise (avocado and oil based)

- Pinch of Pepper
- 1 tsp Sriracha
- 1 tbsp grated Sheep Cheese

Directions:

1. Combine the eggs and water in the Instant Pot. Close the lid and cook on MANUAL for 6 minutes.
2. Perform a quick pressure release and let cool before peeling.
3. Whisk together the sour cream, mayonnaise, pepper, chili powder, and sriracha.
4. Cut the eggs in half and top with the mixture. Sprinkle the cheese over.

Hardboiled Eggs

(Prep + Cook Time: 10 minutes / Servings: 6)

Ingredients:

- 6 Eggs
- 1 ½ cups Water

Directions:

1. Pour the water in your Instant Pot and add the eggs.
2. Close the lid and set the Pressure Release to Sealing.
3. Set the cooker to MANUAL and cook for 6 minutes.
4. Release the pressure naturally, for 10 minutes.
5. Place the eggs in an ice bath for 2 minutes. Peel and serve.

Tempeh Sandwiches

(Prep + Cook Time: 30 minutes / Servings: 4)

Ingredients:

- 12 ounces Tempeh, sliced
- 6 Brioche Buns
- 1 tsp minced Ginger
- 2 tbsp Brown Mustard
- 2 tsp Stevia Brown Sugar
- 1 tsp minced Garlic
- ½ tsp Smoked Paprika
- ½ cup Apple Cider Vinegar
- ⅓ cup Veggie Stock
- 2 tbsp Tamari
- Salt and Pepper, to taste

Directions:

1. Coat the Instant Pot with cooking spray and sauté the tempeh on SAUTÉ for a few minutes.
2. Stir in the remaining ingredients, except the buns, and close the lid. Cook for 2 minutes on MANUAL mode.
3. Do a quick pressure release. Divide the mixture between the buns.

Chef's Selection

Veal and Mushrooms

(Prep + Cook Time: 45 minutes / Servings: 4)

Ingredients:

- 2 pounds Veal Shoulder, cut into chunks
- 16 ounces Shallots, chopped
- 10 ounces Beef Stock
- 8 ounces Mushrooms, sliced
- 3 ½ tbsp Olive Oil
- 2 tbsp Chives, chopped
- 2 ounces White Wine
- 1 tsp minced Garlic
- 1 tbsp Almond Flour
- 1 tsp Sage

Directions:

1. Heat 1 ½ tbsp oil in your Instant Pot selecting SAUTÉ. Add veal and coat with flour. Cook until browned.
2. Add the rest of the oil and cook the mushrooms for 3 minutes.
3. Stir in onions and garlic and cook for 2 minutes.
4. Pour the wine, stock, and sage.
5. Close the lid and cook on MANUAL for 20 minutes at high pressure.
6. Release the pressure naturally for 10 minutes before turning steam valve to Venting to Quick Release remaining pressure. Serve hot.

Chicken Liver Pate

(Prep + Cook Time: 15 minutes / Servings: 16)

Ingredients:

- 1 pound Chicken Livers
- 1 cup chopped Leek
- ⅓ cup Rum
- 2 tsp Olive Oil
- 2 tbsp Ghee Butter
- 1 tbsp Sage
- 1 tsp Basil
- 1 tsp Thyme
- 3 Anchovies

Directions:

1. Heat the oil in your Instant Pot on SAUTÉ and cook the leeks for a few minutes. Add the liver and cook for 3 minutes.
2. Stir in the rum and close the lid. Select MANUAL and cook for 10 minutes. Release the pressure naturally, for 10 minutes.
3. Stir in the remaining ingredients. Transfer to a food processor and pulse until smooth.

Eggs de Provence

(Prep + Cook Time: 20 minutes / Servings: 4)

Ingredients:

- 8 Eggs
- 1 cup Organic Heavy Cream
- 2 Shallots, chopped
- 1 ¼ cups Bacon de Provence, cooked and crumbled
- 1 ½ cups chopped Kale
- 1 tbsp mixed Herbs by choice
- Salt and Pepper, to taste
- 4 tbsp Water

Directions:

1. Whisk the eggs with the water and cream in a baking dish.
2. Stir in the shallots, bacon, kale, and herbs. Season with salt and pepper.
3. Cover with a piece of foil. Pour 1 ½ cups of water in the Instant Pot and lower the trivet. Place the dish inside.
4. Close the lid and cook on MANUAL for 18 minutes at high pressure.
5. When cooking is completes, immediately turn steam vent to Venting to Quick Release pressure. Serve immediately.

Whole Hog Omelet

(Prep + Cook Time: 40 minutes / Servings: 4)

Ingredients:

- 6 Eggs, beaten
- 1 cup shredded Sheep Cheese
- ½ cup diced Ham
- 1 cup ground Sausage
- 4 Bacon Slices, cooked and crumbled
- ½ cup Coconut Milk
- 2 Green Onions, chopped
- Salt and Pepper, to taste

Directions:

1. Whisk all the ingredients together. Transfer to a baking dish.
2. Pour 1 ½ cups water in your Instant Pot and lower the trivet.
3. Place the dish inside the cooker. Close the lid and cook for 20 minutes on MANUAL.
4. Release the pressure naturally, for 10 minutes, and serve.

Cheese and Prosciutto Eggs

(Prep + Cook Time: 10 minutes / Servings: 4)

Ingredients:

- 8 Eggs
- 8 Prosciutto Slices
- 4 Sheep Cheese Slices
- 4 tbsp chopped Spring Onions
- 2 tbsp chopped Parsley
- 2 tbsp Ghee Butter
- 1 tablespoon thinly sliced fresh chives

Directions:

1. Pour 1 ½ cups water in your Instant Pot and lower the trivet.
2. Coat 4 ramekins with the butter.
3. Break 2 eggs into each ramekin and top with the spring onions.
4. Place 2 prosciutto slice over the onions and top with ½ slice of cheese.
5. Sprinkle the parsley over. Cover the ramekins with foil and place them in the Instant Pot. Close the lid and cook for 6 minutes on MANUAL.
6. Once the cooking has completed, set steam vent to Venting to quick-release pressure.
7. Garnish with chives.

Easy Duck with and Ginger

(Prep + Cook Time: 50 minutes / Servings: 8)

Ingredients:

- 1 Duck, chopped into pieces
- 1-inch Ginger, chopped
- 1 tbsp White Wine
- 2 cups Water
- Salt and Pepper, to taste

Directions:

1. Place all of the ingredients in your Instant Pot.
2. Season with salt and pepper to taste.
3. Close the lid and cook on MANUAL for 40 minutes at high pressure.
4. Release the pressure naturally for 5 minutes, and serve immediately.

Vegan Holiday Roast

(Prep + Cook Time: 20 minutes / Servings: 8)

Ingredients:

- 1 Field Roast (such as Hazelnut Cranberry Roast En Croute)
- 1 cup Vegetable Broth
- 1 Celery Stalk, chopped
- 1 Onion, diced
- 2 tsp minced Garlic
- Salt and Pepper, to taste
- 1 ½ tbsp Olive Oil

Directions:

1. Press SAUTÉ on your pressure cooker. Heat the oil in the pot. Cook and stir the onion and celery until soft, about 3 minutes.
2. Add garlic and cook for one more minute; add roast and broth.
3. Close the lid and turn steam valve to sealing. Press MANUAL and cook for 10 minutes at higth pressure.
4. Once cooking is complete, allow pressure to release naturally for 10 minutes before turning steam valve to Venting to Quick Release remaining pressure.
5. Season with salt and pepper before serving.

White Wine Mussels

(Prep + Cook Time: 15 minutes / Servings: 4)

Ingredients:

- 1 Onion, chopped
- 2 pounds Mussels, cleaned
- ½ cup White Wine
- 1 Garlic Clove, crushed
- ½ cup Water
- 1 bunch fresh coriander to garnish

Directions:

1. Heat the oil in pressure cooker set to Sauté. Lay onion and garlic into the oil and cook and stir until soft, about 3 minutes.
2. Add wine and cook for 1 more minute. Place the mussels into the steamer basket on the rack, placing them rounded-side up to fit as many as possible.
3. Lower rack into the cooker and place steamer basket on the rack.
4. Close the lid in place and set steam vent to Sealing. Select MANUAL and cook for 2 minutes on low pressure.
5. Let pressure release naturally for about 10 minutes.
6. Tumble mussels into the steaming liquid in the pot to coat with the wine mixture before serving.
7. Garnish with some freshly chopped coriander.

Buttery and Lemony Dill Clams

(Prep + Cook Time: 10 minutes / Servings: 4)

Ingredients:

- 28 scrubbed Clams
- 1 tbsp minced Dill
- ¼ cup Water
- ½ cup White Wine

- 3 tbsp Lemon Juice
- 2 tbsp Stevia Brown Sugar
- 1 tsp minced Garlic

Directions:

1. Combine all of the ingredients in the Instant Pot and add the clams inside. Close the lid and cook on MANUAL for 5 minutes.
2. Let pressure to release naturally for 5 minutes, then set steam vent to Venting to quick-release remaining pressure. Serve immediately.

Pork Liver and Spring Onion Pate

(Prep + Cook Time: 25 minutes / Servings: 10)

Ingredients:

- 1 pound Pork Liver, chopped
- 4 Spring Onions, chopped
- 2 tbsp Oil
- 4 Garlic Cloves, sliced
- 3 tbsp Almond Flour
- 1 tsp Basil
- Salt and Pepper, to taste

Directions:

1. Heat the oil in your Instant Pot on SAUTÉ. Brown the liver for about 3 minutes. Stir in the remaining ingredients and cook for another minute.
2. Pour a little bit of water to cover. Close the lid.
3. Press MANUAL and cook for 15 minutes. Release the pressure naturally fo 10 minutes.
4. Transfer the mixture to a food processor and pulse until smooth.

Hassle-Free Holiday Roast

(Prep + Cook Time: 75 minutes / Servings: 8)

Ingredients:

- 3 pounds Beef Roast
- 2 cups Beef Broth
- 1 cup chopped Onions
- 2 tsp Olive Oil
- Salt and Pepper, to taste

Directions:

1. Season the meat with salt and pepper.
2. Heat the oil in your Instant Pot by selecting SAUTÉ on High. Add the onion and cook until soft, about 2-3 minutes.
3. Add roast and sear on all sides. Press Cancel to stop Sauté. Pour the broth over and close the lid. Cook for 3 hours on SLOW cook mode.
4. Carve meat and arrange onto a serving platter. Drizzle sauce over roast before serving.

Quail and Pancetta

(Prep + Cook Time: 30 minutes / Servings: 4)

Ingredients:

- 2 Quails, cleaned
- ½ cup Champagne
- 4 ounces Pancetta, chopped
- 2 Scallions, chopped
- ½ Fennel Bulb, chopped
- 1 tsp Thyme
- 1 tsp Rosemary
- Juice of 1 Lemon
- 1 tbsp Olive Oil
- minced flat-leaf Italian parsley to garnish
- Salt and Pepper, to taste

Directions:

1. Add the fennel in the Instant Pot and add 2 cups of water. Cook on MANUAL for 2 minutes. Transfer to a plate and reserve the broth.
2. Heat the oil in the Instant Pot, select SAUTÉ and cook the scallions, pancetta, and all the herbs about 2-3 minutes. Add the quail and brown on all sides, 3 to 5 minutes per side.
3. Pour the broth and champagne over. Season with salt and black pepper to taste. Close the lid in place and turn steam vent handle to Sealing. Select MANUAL and cook for 10 minutes on higth pressure.
4. Let pressure release naturally for 10 minutes, then turn steam vent handle to Venting to quick-release remaining pressure.
5. Garnish with minced parsley, and serve.

Party Crab Legs

(Prep + Cook Time: 20 minutes / Servings: 4)

Ingredients:

- 1 ½ pounds frozen Crab Legs
- 2 tbsp melted Ghee Butter
- 1 cup Veggie Broth
- ½ cup White Wine

Directions:

1. Pour the broth and wine into the Instant Pot.
2. Tumble the crab legs into the steamer basket.
3. Lower rack into the cooker and place steamer basket on the rack.
4. Close the lid and set valve to Sealing.
5. Cook for 4 minutes on STEAM at high pressure.
6. When cooking time is up, do a quick pressure release.
7. Serve the crab legs on a platter drizzled with butter.

Party Duck Bites

(Prep + Cook Time: 25 minutes / Servings: 6)

Ingredients:

- 1 ½ pounds Duck, cut up
- ⅓ cup Tomato Puree
- 1 ½ cups Water
- 2 tsp Basil
- Salt and Pepper, to taste

Sauce:

- ⅓ cup Organ Sour Cream
- ½ cup chopped Parsley
- ¼ cup Olive Oil
- 2 tbsp Lemon Juice
- 2 Jalapenos, chopped
- 1 Garlic Clove

Directions:

1. Pour the water in the Instant Pot and place the trivet in the water. Place the duck a baking pan; stir in all duck ingredients.
2. Close the lid and cook on MANUAL for 15 minutes at high pressure.
3. Once the cooking is complete, set steam vent to Venting to quick-release pressure.
4. Blend the all the sauce ingredients with an immersion blender until smooth and transfer to a small serving bowl.
5. Toss the duck in the sauce and serve immediately.

Festive Rosemary Chicken

(Prep + Cook Time: 55 minutes / Servings: 4)

Ingredients:

- 1 Whole Chicken
- 1 tbsp Cayenne Pepper
- 2 Rosemary Sprigs
- 2 Garlic Cloves, crushed
- ¼ Onion
- 1 tsp dried Rosemary
- Salt and Pepper, to taste
- 1 ½ cups Chicken Broth

Directions:

1. Wash and pat dry the chicken. Season with salt, pepper, rosemary, and cayenne pepper. Rub the spices well into the meat.
2. Place the onion, garlic, and rosemary sprig inside the chicken's cavity.
3. Place the chicken in the Instant Pot. Pour the broth around the chicken (not over). Cook for 30 minutes on MEAT/STEW at high pressure.
4. Once cooking is complete, use a natural release. This will take 10 to 15 minutes.
5. Let stand 5-10 minutes, before carving. Serve with vegetables.

Fancy Shrimp Scampi

(Prep + Cook Time: 45 minutes / Servings: 4)

Ingredients:

- 2 tbsp Ghee Butter
- 1 tbsp grated Sheep Cheese
- 2 Shallots, chopped
- ¼ cup White Wine
- 1 tsp minced Garlic
- 2 tbsp Lemon Juice
- 1 pound Shrimp, peeled and deveined
- Extra chopped parsley for garnishing

Directions:

1. Melt the butter in the Instant Pot on SAUTÉ and cook the shallots until soft, about 2-3 minutes. Add garlic and cook for 1 more minute.
2. Stir in the wine and cook for another minute. Press Cancel.
3. Add the remaining ingredients except the cheese and stir to combine.
4. Close the lid, select MANUAL and cook for 2 minutes at high pressure.
5. Release the pressure naturally for about 10 minutes.
6. Serve immediately sprinkled with some sheep cheese and chopped parsley.

Made in the USA
Middletown, DE
20 August 2018